MELALEUCA ESSENTIAL OIL:

The Ultimate Guide to Get Amazing Results of Tea Tree Oil

James Amelia

Copy Right© 2019
James Amelia

This publication may not be reproduced, distributed or transmitted by any means without the prior written consent of the author first had and obtained. The facts herein provided is truthful in all its entirety and coherent, in that no legal responsibility, in the form of consideration or else by the use or misuse of any strategies, procedures or directions contained within shall lie against the author such liability thereon is the sole and the utter obligation of the reader solely. Under no situation will any legal duty or blames be imputed or held out unfavorable the publisher(s) for any form of compensation, damages, pecuniary loss due to the information contained herein be it direct or indirect.

The material offered here is for the purposes of information only and is universal as such. The information presented here is without any form of contract or guarantee or indemnity whether with the reader or any third party. Consult your doctor before the application of any procedure herein.

TABLE OF CONTENTS

CHAPTER 1 — 1

Tea Tree Essential Oil 1
Contents of Tea Tree Oil 2

CHAPTER 2 — 5

Benefits of Tea Tree Essential Oil For The Skin 5
TTO for Longer and Thicker Hair 5
How to use Tea Tree Oil for Dandruff Treatment 7
TTO as Natural Moisturizers 8
How to use TTO 10
How to Use TTO to treat Head Lice 13
Treatment of Acne with Tea Tree Oil 14
How to Use TTO in Treating Acne 15
How to use TTO to Treat Eczema and psoriasis 16
How to use TTO 17
Effective Means of Controlling Gland that produces Skin Oil 19
How to use TTO to Treat Stye 20

How to use Tea Tree Oil for the Treatment of Belly Button Infections 21
How to use TTO to Heal/Dry socket pains 22
How to Prepare and Use TTO to Control Body Odour 23
How to use Tea Tree oil as Room Spray 25

CHAPTER 3   27

You Can Make TTO At Home 27

CHAPTER 4   30

Tips and Tricks for Using TTO 30

CHAPTER 5   34

Dosages of Tea Tree Oil 34
Side effects of Tea Tree Oil 36
How to Buy Tea Tree Oil Online 37
Glossary 38

CHAPTER 1

Tea Tree Essential Oil

Melaleuca alternitolia, is a rich source of Tea Tree Oil (TTO for short as I will refer to this short abbreviation in this book, whenever I make reference to tea tree oil), a native of New South Wales and Queensland, Australia, it has become so popular today due to its versatile usage. Tea Tree Oil is also an essential oil that possesses very virile antibacterial properties and can treat many infections.

The Aboriginals have employed the use of TTO as medicine for many centuries. The leaves are pulverised by the aborigines and the oil extracted which is mostly inhaled for the treatment of coughs, cold, and skin related diseases.

At present, tea tree oil is used today as one hundred percent undiluted or clean oil. There are also diluted forms of TTO which are in use today.

Contents of Tea Tree Oil

The first compound that is found in TTO is Terpinen 4 01, which has been proven to destroy fungi, bacteria, and some types of viruses. Surprisingly, Terpinen 4 ol, has been known to raise the activity of white blood cells which also helps in fighting germs and other alien invaders. As a result of this anti-germs property which TTO possess, it has become very valuable in the treatment of many skin related conditions and infections.

Tea Tree Oil: How Does It work?

Tea tree oil can be termed an essential oil with fresh camphor smell. Derived from the leaves of Melaleuca alternifolia, commonly found in Queensland and New South Wales, Australia. Its tree grows up to 7 meters tall.

The question whether this oil work is important. One reason why the Tea tree oil works is because of its structure and composition. The oil has over 100 components, but the major elements are sesquiterpenes, monoterpenes, and their individual alcohols.

The Benefits of Tea Tree Oil

It has been explained above that TTO has multifarious uses to which the oil can be effectively used for. We will consider some of these uses for skin, hair and for other purposes.

CHAPTER 2

Benefits of Tea Tree Essential Oil For The Skin

TTO for Longer and Thicker Hair

If your hair is short, and you experience frequent breakage of your hair, I present to you your ultimate solution – Tea Tree Oil. Tea Tree Oil can enhance the growth of your hair by unclogging hair follicles and provide nourishment for hair root.

How to use TTO for Longer and Thicker Hair

To use Tea Tree Oil for the purposes of making your hair thicker and stronger, simply apply the oil to your hair by spraying it. Fill your bottle of glass spray with enough quantity of water and add 5 drops of TTO for every ounce. Then spray it in the morning and allow it throughout the day for hair growth.

Effective Remedy for Dandruff

Due to the high presence of antibacterial and fungi properties, TTO is ideal for the treating of dandruff. The Tea tree oil battles the fungi that cause dandruff without necessarily drying your hair scalp. Besides it ability to kill dandruff, TTO serves as a good natural conditioner that prevents issues that causes scalp flake

How to use Tea Tree Oil for Dandruff Treatment

If you want to treat dandruff with TTO, add normal shampoo to hair approximately ten drops for every eight ounces of shampoo. Before washing your hair, make sure that you allow the shampoo and the TTO to mix well for at least 5 minutes. If you desire faster and quicker results from the use of TTO for the treatment of dandruff, use it overnight. Just add a ¾ bottle of olive oil, almond oil, coconut oil, jojoba oil, etc. After that, add 15 drops of TTO and blend it. Apply it to your hair scalp and massage it for some few minutes and ensure that your scalp is wholly saturated.

TTO as Natural Moisturizers

Tea Tree oil has amazing benefits because of its ability to nourish and moisturize your dry scalp. It clears any blockage in your pores and prevents dry hair.

How to use TTO as Moisturizers

Mix a few droplets of jojoba oil with TTO and massage the mix for about 15 minutes. Rinse it very well and wash your hair. Carry out this process as regularly as you can. It can also stop itchy hair. Add shampoo to your hair and add a few droplets of your normal hair conditioner. Blend it well and add it to your scalp. Allow it some few minutes before washing.

Hair Cleanser

Tea Tree oil performs various hair functions. It can be used as your regular shampoo at home for your hair.

How to use Tea Tree oil as your hair cleanser

Add some few droplets of Tea Tree oil to your normal shampoo. By doing so, it gives your shampoo added therapeutic elements. Apply the mix to your hair scalp and massage it for some time. After that, rinse it very well.

Treating Dry and Itchy Hair

This is another amazing benefit of using Tea Tree oil for your hair. It can be used to treat dry and itchy hair. You will need any carrier, that is, any oil of your choice such as jojoba oil, almond oil, or sesame oil. Since Tea tree oil destroys microbes that are known for causing damage to the scalp, it calms your itchy scalp and subsequently heals it. The common causes of itchiness are dirty scalp, dandruff, and dryness.

How to use TTO to Heal Dry and Itchy Hair

Using your carrier, (olive oil, Jojoba, almond, or sesame oil) add at least two droplets of TTO to half a cup of your carrier

Tea Tree Oil

oil. It is advisable to use little quantity of TTO if your hair is naturally oily, and a higher quantity if your hair is naturally dry. Warm your oil mix. Heat normal water on the stove. Before the water boils, remove the pot from the stove and set your oil in a separate vessel. Put your oil into the warm water until the oil becomes warm. Pour the oil on your wrist in order to feel the temperature of the oil so that it is not excessively hot. Divide the oil into 4 sections for easy distribution of the oil. You can make use of an applicator to apply the oil to all parts of your hair. Massage the oil mix into your hair scalp carefully. Now, cover your hair using a plastic shower cap and allow it for 30 minutes.

James Amelia

<u>Head Lice Treatment</u>

Tea Tree oil has been shown through various studies to destroy lice that are in their nymph and adult phases of life. It also decreases the number of eggs hatched by lice. Research also shows that ¼ children that were treated using chemical anti lice shampoo that contains pyrethrins and piperonyl butoxide were later free of lice. On the other hand, almost all the children that were treated with TTO were completely free from lice. The TTO can easily dissolve the sticky texture that links the nits to the shaft of your hair.

Tea Tree Oil

How to Use TTO to treat Head Lice

In a moderate bowl, combine 3 -4 droplets of shampoo and 3-4 droplets of lavender essential oil and mix it very well. Then add a quarter shampoo and mix it very well. Pour a little drop of extra virgin olive oil. This will help in suffocating the lice. Pour the shampoo mix into your hair and massage the scalp area very well. Put a shower cap on your hair and cover it for at least 30 minutes. Use your hands on your hair to remove the lice. Rinse it well. If you desire, you can apply hair conditioner for easy removal of the lice. Comb your hair so that the lice can be removed. Do this frequently for the next 7 days for all the nits, and the lice to be removed.

Tea Tree Oil for Skin

Treatment of Acne with Tea Tree Oil

Acne is a skin disorder characterized by black, red, or white pimples on the skin surface, particularly on the face of individuals suffering from it, which is caused largely due to the inflammation or sebaceous glands that are infected. This skin condition is common among adolescents. However, no matter how bad the acne may be, there is a good treatment that will heal acne completely through the use of Tea tree oil. As we have stated before, that TTO has antibacterial elements which help in dealing with acne. A simple 5 percent solution of TTO performs just like the majority of the popular acne drugs such as benzoyl peroxide.

How to Use TTO in Treating Acne

Dilute a little drop of Tea Tree Oil with about 20 -40 droplets of witch hazel. Apply it to the skin surface once or twice daily using a cotton swab. You should do this cautiously as excessive use of TTO can dry your skin and make your own body to produce its oil which will make your acne worse.

Treatment for Eczema and Psoriasis

This is one of the great functions performed by TTO. It can be used for the treatment of Psoriasis and eczema.

How to use TTO to Treat Eczema and psoriasis

Mix a teaspoon of coconut oil and five droplets of TTO and another five droplets of lavender oil to produce a home-made TTO eczema lotion or any body soap.

<u>Treatment of Minor Cuts and Infections</u>

Tea Tree oil can also be used to treat minor cut and infections when it is mixed with lavender oil. It advisable to thoroughly clean the cut or infection with hydrogen peroxide or water. Then apply the TTO and properly cover the infection or cut.

Tea Tree Oil

<u>Treat Ringworm</u>

Tea Tree oil, being antifungal in nature can easily treat ringworm.

Before usage, you have to wash the area that is affected by the ringworm very well. To prevent contamination, any clothing that you use to dry the affected place must be put in the washing machine.

How to use TTO for Ringworm Treatment.

Sterilize your cotton swab and then add some few drops of oil to the end of the cotton swab. After that, apply the swab to the affected places. Perform this procedure three times daily for maximum results.

Removal of Makeup

You can use TTO to remove makeup from your face. To use it, get canola oil of a least ¼ cup and mix it with 10 drops of TTO in a 4 ounce glass jar that has been sterilized and shake it so that it mixes very well. Store it in a cold, dry place for use.

Treatment of Cold sores and Zap boils

If you want to use TTO to treat cold sores and zap boils, apply it directly to the cold sore. This should be done at least three to four times every day. Tea Tree oil can be used to treat staph infection, especially those have proven resistant to many antibiotic.

Tea Tree Oil

<u>Soothes Athletes Foot</u>

Tea Tree oil has been shown to treat athlete foot from burning, sealing, inflammation, and itching. If you are an athlete and you feel any of the above listed conditions, TTO can serve as a good means of treatment.

Effective Means of Controlling Gland that produces Skin Oil

Over production of sebum is one of the main causes of acne and dandruff. One of the main works that TTO does is to control skin oil production. Once it controls skin oil production, acne and dandruff will be prevented.

Treatment of Stye

Tea Tree Oil can be used to treat a stye, an inflamed swelling that occurs at the edge of the eyelid. A stye is often caused by bacterial infection. Since TTO possesses anti-bacterial properties, it is a good means of treatment. What the oil does is to decrease inflammation and bacterial activity.

How to use TTO to Treat Stye

Mix one teaspoon of TTO and 2 teaspoonfuls of water. The water should be properly filtered. Mix the two together and store it in a refrigerator. Carefully apply it around the eye three times each day until the pain, and the swelling disappears.

Tea Tree Oil

<u>Treating Belly Buttons Related Infections</u>

We have stated earlier that TTO has antibacterial and fungi elements. As a result of these properties, TTO can serve as a good treatment for belly buttons infections.

How to use Tea Tree Oil for the Treatment of Belly Button Infections

Mix 4-5 droplets of TTO with a teaspoon of olive oil or coconut oil. Use a neat cotton ball and gently apply the oil to the affected place. Allow it for 10 minutes and thereafter clean it off using a neat tissue. Do this for about three times each day until you begin to see results?

Healing of Dry Socket Pains

Dry socket pains, mostly experienced by individuals whose teeth have been removed can be treated with TTO due to its antiseptic properties. This can also be used to prevent tooth infection.

How to use TTO to Heal/Dry socket pains

Add two droplets of melt swab. Apply it to the affected place and let it remain for 5 minutes. Remove the cotton swap and rinse it with warm water. Carry out this procedure for 2 to 3 times every day.

Heal Blisters

You can use TTO to treat blisters.

Mix your TTO with plain or vegetable oil. Use a neat cotton ball and apply it to the affected place. It should stay for about 10 minutes before rinsing it with cold water.

<u>Effective control of Body odor</u>

If you are suffering from armpit odor, TTO can be used to control it owing to the presence of antibacterial properties. Since sweat does not smell, but rather the combination with bacterial that cause it to smell, then the antibacterial in TTO can serve as a deodorant and effectively control arm pit odour.

How to Prepare and Use TTO to Control Body Odour

Ingredients

3 tablespoons of coconut oil

3 tablespoons of shea butter

¼ cup of cornstarch

¼ cup of baking soda

About 20-30 Droplets of Tea Tree oil

Instruction

Melt coconut oil, shea butter in a moderate glass jar. Remove jar from heat when it has melted and pour in cornstarch, TTO, and baking soda. Wait for several hours for the mixture to be ready. Once it is ready, pour it into container/deodorant stick for use.

Use your finger to rub it under your armpit like a lotion.

Tea Tree Oil

Use as Diffuser and Room Spray

Tea tree oil can be used as air spray for the purpose of disinfecting rooms and nontoxic spay for removing bacteria and mold in the environment.

How to use Tea Tree oil as Room Spray

What you need:

4 Drops of Tea Tree oil

4 drops of Peppermint essential oil

4 Drops of lemon essential oil

4 drops of Eucalyptus essential oil

Now, mix all these oils before you combine them in a 2 ml glass bottle and roll bottle in between your hands for proper blending.

CHAPTER 3

You Can Make TTO At Home

If you don't want to purchase tea tree oil from online, you can make your own tea tree oil.

<u>Ingredients</u>

A Bunch of tea tree leaves

Instructions

Pour a bunch of tea tree leaves in a pot. Cover the leaves with water. Set your vegetable steamer in a pot. Insert measuring cup in the steamer.

Cover the pot. Let the knob nub of your cover points in the direction of your measuring cup. Boil the water so that you can steam the leaves. Allow water to condense and eventually evaporate. The condensation is necessary so that it will slide to the handle and into your measuring cup.

Put 4 ice cubes on the top of the overturned cover/lid for rapid condensation of the steam. When the ice melt, put off the heat.

Tea Tree Oil

Take off your lid and empty the ice cube water into your kitchen sink. Take off your glass measuring cup.

Pour the substance into your measuring cup into a separation funnel. Seal the top of your funnel and then shake it thoroughly.

Overturn your funnel and open for the purpose of releasing the pressure in it. When you do this, the oil will easily float on the top of the water.

Place a glass bottle under your stopcock and discharge the water. Pour your oil into a coloured glass bottle.

Repeat this procedure for about three times for extracting all the oil from the leaves.

CHAPTER 4

Tips and Tricks for Using TTO

Tips 1#: Excessive Drops

Never use excessive droplets of Tea Tree Oil as only a few drops will be sufficient with your carrier. When using your shampoo or conditioner, add 10 drops of TTO for each ounce of shampoo. When TTO is excessively used, it can lead to weak hair and other hair damages.

Tips 2#: Tough Dandruff

The reason why we employ the use of tea tree oil is simple. There are certain types of difficult and tough dandruff that shampoo may not deal with. It requires other forms of tougher measures; Tea Tree oil is one of those tougher measures. So when shampoo fails, ensure that you add a few drops of TTO with your carrier and be sure to see dandruff vanish within the shortest possible time.

Tips 3#: No Limitation

Tea Tree oil can be used for any type of hair texture. So whether your hair is short, small, tough, or, soft TTO can still be used with amazing results for your hair.

Tips 4#: Diluting Tea Tree Oil

Tea Tree Oil is strong that is why it has to be dissolved into another hair carrier such as olive oil, coconut oil, jojoba oil, etc., prior to applying it to your hair scalp. Whenever TTO is applied without diluting, it can lead to irritation and cause itchiness or even dryness. The moment you noticed irritation, dryness or itchiness, stop using TTO.

Tips 5#: Product Tip

As a result of its multiple functions, many products have incorporated some percentages of TTO in their products such as hair conditioners and shampoo. It is only when you use it that you can know what works for you.

CHAPTER 5

Dosages of Tea Tree Oil

There is a recommended dosage of Tea Tree Oil.

<u>Dosage For Adult</u>

Acne: 5% TTO gel applied every day.

Infected eyelashes: Scrub the eyelid every week with 50% TTO and combine it everyday scrubs of the affected eyelid with Tea Tree Shampoo or 10% TTO. It should be applied once/twice daily for approximately 3 to 5 minutes for 6 weeks.

Nail fungus: 100% TTO solution that should be applied twice every day for the period of 6 months.

Athlete's foot: 25%/50% TTO solution that should be applied two times daily for at least 1 month.

<u>Children Dosage</u>

Acne: 5% TTO gel applied every day.

Infected eyelashes: scrub the affected eyelid every week with 50% TTO and everyday eyelid massages using about 5% of tea tree ointment

Side effects of Tea Tree Oil

<u>Toxicity</u>

Tea Tree Oil is very toxic when consumed orally. Whenever the oil is applied orally, it can lead to serious complications.

<u>Skin Irritation and swelling</u>

Tea tree oil may result in skin swelling and irritation in certain people. The oil can lead to dryness and itchiness in some people.

<u>Hormonal Problems</u>

When you use tea tree oil on the skin surface of young boys that have not yet attained the age of puberty, it can cause hormone imbalance. There are cases where boys begin to develop breast because of the TTO.

<u>Mouthwash problems</u>

When using Tea tree oil to gargle or wash your mouth, you need to be careful because the strong substances in tea tree oil have been shown to cause serious injury to oversensitive membranes in the gullet.

How to Buy Tea Tree Oil Online

There are various places that you can purchase Tea Tree oil online, but the popular ones are:

Amazon.com

Walmart.com

Glossary

A

Acne, 3, 10, 11, 26, 27
almond oil, 6, 8
Athlete's foot, 27

C

coconut oil, 6, 12, 16, 18, 24
conditioner, 5, 7, 10, 23

D

Dandruff, 3, 5, 23
Diffuser, 4, 19

E

Eczema, 3, 12
essential, 1, 2, 10, 19

H

hair, 3, 4, 5, 6, 7, 8, 9, 10, 23, 24, 25
Hair, 3, 4, 5, 7
hydrogen peroxide, 12

I

Infected eyelashes, 26, 27

J

jojoba oil, 6, 8, 24

L

Lice, 3, 9, 10

Tea Tree Oil

M

makeup, 13
Makeup, 4, 13
Melaleuea, 1
moisturize, 6
Moisturizers, 3, 6

O

Oil, 4, 1, 4, 14

R

Rinse, 6, 10

S

scalp, 5, 6, 7, 8, 9, 10, 24
shampoo, 5, 7, 9, 10, 23, 24, 25
skin, 2, 3, 10, 11, 15, 28
Skin, 3, 4, 5, 4, 10, 14, 28

T

Tea Tree Oil, 1

Tea Tree Oil, 1, 3, 4, 5, 1, 2, 3, 4, 5, 6, 8, 10, 11, 13, 15, 16, 20, 23, 24, 26, 27, 29
terpinen, 2
Treat, 3, 4, 12, 13, 15
Treatment, 1, 3, 4, 9, 10, 12, 13, 14, 15, 16

U

Uses, 3

James Amelia

www.ingramcontent.com/pod-product-compliance
Lightning Source LLC
Chambersburg PA
CBHW030536220526
45463CB00007B/2863